Everything You Need to Know About Birth Defects

Causes ◆ Symptoms ◆ Treatment

Watch a video version:

https://www.youtube.com/watch?v=lXwfK9Di_KQ

This book is based on information and recommendations by the Department of Health, United States government.

Created By The Bizmove Health Team

Disclaimer

All the content found in this book was created for informational purposes only. The Content is not intended to be a substitute for professional medical advice, diagnosis, or treatment. Always seek the advice of your physician or other qualified health provider with any questions you may have regarding a medical condition. Never disregard professional medical advice or delay in seeking it because of something you have read in this book.

ISBN: 9798747252707

Everything You Need to Know About Birth Defects

Birth defects are structural (how the body is built) or functional (how the body works) abnormalities present at birth that can cause physical disability, intellectual and developmental disorders, and other health problems. This information focuses on structural birth defects, such as heart, limb, or brain malformations, their causes, their prevention, and their treatments.

Researchers have identified thousands of different birth defects, and some are more disruptive than others. If not detected and treated quickly, some can be fatal or cause lifelong disabilities. Currently, the Centers for Disease Control and Prevention notes that birth defects are the leading cause of death for infants during the first year of life.

Understanding human development across the lifespan, including birth defects and related or resulting disabilities, was a primary reason NICHD was established. The Institute is a leader in research on birth defects, their causes, their prevention and treatments, and their long-term health outcomes.

NICHD is aware that the term "birth defects" carries negative undertones and that the term does not reflect the many abilities and talents of those affected by these problems. Communities are discussing alternative terms for describing these birth problems. Until a consensus is reached, this website uses the term "birth defects" to describe these health issues.

About Birth Defects

Birth defects are structural or functional abnormalities present at birth that can cause physical disability, intellectual and developmental disability (IDD), and other health problems. Some may be fatal, especially if not detected and treated early.

There are two main categories of birth defects: structural birth defects and functional/developmental birth defects. This information focuses on structural birth defects, their causes, their prevention, and their treatment. Functional/developmental birth defects are addressed more completely in the IDDs content.

Some birth defects affect many parts or processes in the body, leading to both structural and functional problems.

Researchers have identified thousands of different birth defects. According to the Centers for Disease Control and Prevention (CDC), birth defects are the leading cause of death for infants in the United States during the first year of life.

What are the types of birth defects?

There are two main categories of birth defects.

Structural Birth Defects

Structural birth defects are related to a problem with the structure of body parts. These can include:

- Cleft lip or cleft palate
- Heart defects, such as missing or misshaped valves
- Abnormal limbs, such as a clubfoot
- Neural tube defects, such as spina bifida, and problems related to the growth and development of the brain and spinal cord

Functional or Developmental Birth Defects

Functional or developmental birth defects are related to a problem with how a body part or body system works or functions. These problems can include:

- **Nervous system or brain problems.** These include intellectual and developmental disabilities, behavioral disorders, speech or language difficulties, seizures, and movement trouble. Some examples of birth defects that affect the nervous system include Down syndrome, Prader-Willi syndrome, and Fragile X syndrome.
- **Sensory problems.** Examples include hearing loss and visual problems, such as blindness or deafness.
- **Metabolic disorders.** These involve problems with certain chemical reactions in the body, such as conditions that limit the body's ability to rid itself of waste materials or harmful chemicals. Two common metabolic disorders are phenylketonuria and hypothyroidism.
- **Degenerative disorders.** These are conditions that might not be obvious at birth but cause one or more aspects of health to steadily get worse. Examples of degenerative disorders are muscular dystrophy and X-linked adrenoleukodystrophy, which leads to problems of the nervous system and the adrenal glands and was the subject of the movie "Lorenzo's Oil."

Some birth defects affect many parts or processes in the body, leading to both structural and functional problems.

This information focuses on structural birth defects, their causes, their prevention, and their treatment. Functional/developmental birth defects are addressed more completely in the intellectual and developmental disabilities content.

How many people are affected by/at risk for birth defects?

CDC estimates that birth defects occur in about 1 in every 33 infants born in the United States each year.

Birth defects can occur during any pregnancy, but some factors increase the risk for birth defects. The following situations place pregnant women at higher risk of having a child with a birth defect:

- **Lack of folic acid.** Women who are pregnant or who could become pregnant should take 400 micrograms of folic acid every day to prevent neural tube defects_(NTDs). However, according to the Centers for Disease Control and Prevention (CDC), only 2 out of every 5 women of childbearing age take folic acid every day.
- **Drinking alcohol.**Drinking alcohol during pregnancy can lead to a variety of problems, including birth defects. For example, using alcohol can lead to fetal alcohol syndrome, which is characterized by intellectual or developmental

disability (IDD), physical challenges, and behavioral problems. There is no safe level of alcohol consumption during pregnancy.

- **Smoking cigarettes.** Smoking cigarettes during pregnancy can lead to a variety of problems, including lung problems such as asthma. Evidence also strongly suggests that certain birth defects, such as problems with the heart and intestines, are caused by smoking during pregnancy.
- **Using drugs.** Using drugs during pregnancy can increase the risk of various birth defects, including IDDs and behavioral problems, as well as pregnancy loss and stillbirth.
- **Medication use.** Certain medications are known to cause birth defects if taken during pregnancy. Thalidomide, which is currently used to treat certain cancers and other serious conditions, was once sold as a treatment for morning sickness until it was discovered that it caused severe birth defects. Infants whose mothers took thalidomide had a range of structural and functional problems, including misshapen ears and shortened limbs. Although the thalidomide situation led to much stricter controls on drugs used during pregnancy, the majority of medications currently used by pregnant women have not been tested for safety or efficacy in pregnant women. Addressing this issue is the

primary focus of NICHD's Obstetric-Fetal Pharmacology Research Units Network. Women who are pregnant or who might become pregnant should discuss all medications, both prescription and over-the-counter, and supplements they take with their health care providers.

- **Infections.** Women who get certain infections during pregnancy are at higher risk for having a child with birth defects. Some of the more common infections that are linked to birth defects are cytomegalovirus, a common virus that spreads through body fluids and usually causes no symptoms in healthy people, and toxoplasmosis, a parasitic infection that spreads through contact with cat feces, raw meat, and contaminated food and water. Zika virus infection is linked to microcephaly in newborn babies—a condition in which the brain and skull are smaller than normal. The Pregnancy topic has more information on infections that can cause birth defects and other problems in newborns and on ways to prevent them during pregnancy, and CDC provides tips for preventing infections before and during pregnancy.

- **Obesity or uncontrolled diabetes.** NICHD research found that the risk of newborn heart defects and neural tube defects increased with maternal obesity. Additional NICHD research suggest that children of obese parents may be at risk for developmental delays. Obesity is also associated with other health problems and long-term health issues. Poorly controlled blood sugar places women at higher risk of having a baby who is too large, has breathing problems, or has other poor health outcomes. These outcomes are likely regardless of whether the woman had diabetes before she got pregnant (type 1 or 2 diabetes) or whether she developed diabetes during pregnancy (gestational diabetes).

- **Exposure to things in the environment.** Pregnant women who breathe in, eat, drink, or get things into their bodies in other ways may also be at increased risk of birth defects. For example, pregnant women who are exposed to high levels of radiation, such as cancer treatments, are at higher risk for birth defects in their infants. Handling or breathing in certain chemicals can also increase the risk of birth defects.

What causes birth defects?

Different birth defects have different causes, and the causes of many birth defects remain unknown.

A specific condition might be caused by one or more of the following primary problems:

- **Genetic problems.** One or more genes might have a change or mutation that results in them not working properly, such as in Fragile X syndrome. Similarly, a gene or part of the gene might be missing.
- **Chromosomal problems.** In some cases, a chromosome or part of a chromosome might be missing, such as in Turner syndrome, when a female is missing an X chromosome. Other birth defects result from having an extra chromosome, such as in Klinefelter syndrome and Down syndrome.
- **Infections.** Women who get certain infections during pregnancy are at higher risk for having a child with birth defects. For example, infection with Zika virus during pregnancy is linked with the birth defect called microcephaly, in which the brain and skull are smaller than normal. Zika infection in pregnancy is linked to other structural problems with the brain as well. Our Pregnancy topic has more information on infections that can cause birth defects and other problems in newborns and on ways to prevent them during pregnancy, and CDC provides tips for preventing infections before and during pregnancy.
- **Exposure to medications, chemicals, or other agents during pregnancy.** The infants whose mothers took thalidomide are examples of

an exposure leading to birth defects. Other examples include exposure to rubella (also called German measles) and toxic chemicals, such as hydrocarbons.

How do health care providers diagnose birth defects?

Diagnosis of birth defects depends on the specific problem and parts or systems of the body that are affected.

Many structural problems, such as club foot or cleft palate, are detected and diagnosed after a physical examination of the baby immediately after birth. For other conditions, newborn screening or prenatal testing is the only way to detect and diagnose problems.

This information focuses on structural birth defects, their causes, their prevention, and their treatments. Functional/developmental birth defects are addressed more completely in the intellectual and developmental disabilities content and in condition-specific topics.

Newborn Screening

Newborn screening, a process that tests infants' blood for different health conditions, including many birth defects, provides one method of detecting problems. Newborn screening does not diagnose any specific conditions but detects that a problem may exist. By detecting problems immediately after birth, conditions can be diagnosed and treated before they have lifelong effects.

In addition, newborn screening routinely includes test for hearing problems, as well as pulse oximetry (test of baby's pulse rate and blood oxygen levels) to detect critical congenital heart defects.

Infants who are at high risk for certain conditions—for example, because of their family history—can undergo additional testing at birth to detect these conditions and treat them if needed. This type of screening has been effective in detecting some cases of Menkes disease, allowing for treatment to begin before health problems occur.

Prenatal Screening

During pregnancy, women have routine tests, such as blood and urine tests, to check for diabetes, signs of infection, or disorders of pregnancy such as preeclampsia. Blood tests also measure the levels of certain substances in a woman's blood that determine the risk of the fetus for certain chromosomal disorders and neural tube defects.

Ultrasound screenings, creating a picture using sound, allow providers to view the developing fetus in the womb. Some birth defects, such as spina bifida, are detectable on ultrasounds.

Health care providers recommend that certain pregnant women, including those who are older than 35 years of age and those with a family history of certain conditions, get additional prenatal tests to screen for birth defects. Prenatal detection allows doctors to start treatment as early as possible for some birth defects.

Noninvasive prenatal testing (NIPT).

NIPT is not a routine prenatal test but is used when a routine test suggests that the fetus may have a chromosomal disorder, such as having an extra or missing chromosome in each cell, which occurs in disorders such as Down syndrome, Patau syndrome, and Edwards syndrome.

NIPT analyzes the placental DNA present in the mother's blood; it does not require cell samples from inside the womb.

Currently, experts recommend NIPT only for high-risk pregnancies. This method does not detect open neural tube defects, nor does it predict late pregnancy complications.

Amniocentesis

Amniocentesis (pronounced *am-nee-oh-sen-TEE-sis*) is a test that is usually performed to determine whether a fetus has a genetic disorder. In this test, a doctor takes a small amount of fluid from the womb using a long needle. The fluid, called amniotic (pronounced *am-nee-OT-ik*) fluid, contains cells that have genetic material that is the same as the fetus's genetic material. A laboratory grows the cells and then examines their genetic material for any problems. Some birth defects that can be detected with amniocentesis are Down syndrome and certain types of muscular dystrophy.

There is a slight risk of pregnancy loss with amniocentesis, so women should discuss the procedure with their health care provider before making a decision about the test.

Chorionic Villus Sampling (CVS)

This test extracts cells from inside the womb to determine whether the fetus has a genetic disorder. Using a long needle, the doctor takes cells from the chorionic villi (pronounced *KOHR-ee-on-ik VILL-i*), which are tissues in the placenta, the organ in the womb that nourishes the fetus. The genetic material in the chorionic villus cells is identical to that of the fetal cells.

Like amniocentesis, CVS can be used to test for chromosomal disorders and other genetic problems. CVS can be done earlier in pregnancy than amniocentesis, but it is also associated with a slightly higher risk of miscarriage than amniocentesis. Women who are considering CVS should discuss the test and the risks with her health care provider.

What are the treatments for birth defects?

Because the symptoms and problems caused by birth defects vary, treatments for birth defects also vary. Treatments range from medications and therapies to surgeries and assistive devices.

This information focuses on structural birth defects, their causes, their prevention, and their treatments. Functional/developmental birth defects are addressed more completely in the intellectual and developmental disabilities content and in the condition-specific topics.

For example:

- Steroid medications, such as prednisone, can help people with muscular dystrophy increase muscle strength, ability, and respiratory function and slow the progression of weakness. Physical therapy is also useful for building strength and reducing weakness.

- Infants with cerebral palsy may receive sensory-motor therapy using Velcro-covered "sticky mittens" to help them "snag" and explore objects they are unable to grasp in the hand.
- Assistive devices include orthopedic braces to help patients with limb defects to walk and cochlear implants for hearing impairment.
- In the Management of Myelomeningocele Study (MOMS), conducted through NICHD's Maternal-Fetal Surgery Network, researchers tested a surgical procedure to correct a severe form of spina bifida while the fetus was still in the womb. Although the surgery itself carried risks, it greatly reduced health complications for the infants who received it, including greater likelihood of being able to walk without assistance. Visit http://nichd.nih.gov/news/resources/spotlight/pages/021011-spina-bifida-MOMS.aspx for more information.
- Gene therapy approaches, in which a gene that is mutated or missing is replaced by a normal version of the gene, are being tested for a variety of genetic disorders. Some examples of disorders that are being treated successfully with gene therapy include genetic disorders of the immune system, the muscles, and the eyes. Recent NICHD-supported research on Duchenne muscular dystrophy used genome editing

techniques to improve leg grip strength in a mouse model by "turning on" a gene for a specific protein used in muscles.

Appendix A: Guide to Better Living

Note: Always consult your physician before making any changes to your diet, physical activity or life style.

Is your health condition requires that you make changes to your diet, physical activity, or life style? Are you thinking about being more active? Have you been trying to cut back on less healthy foods? Are you starting to eat better and move more but having a hard time sticking with these changes?

Old habits die hard. Changing your habits is a process that involves several stages. Sometimes it takes a while before changes become new habits. And, you may face roadblocks along the way.

Adopting new, healthier habits may protect you from serious health problems. New habits, like healthy eating and regular physical activity, may also help you manage your weight and have more energy. After a while, if you stick with these changes, they may become part of your daily routine.

The information below outlines four stages you may go through when changing your health habits or behavior. You will also find tips to help you improve your eating, physical activity habits, and overall health. The four stages of changing a health behavior are

- contemplation
- preparation
- action
- maintenance

What stage of change are you in?

Contemplation: "I'm thinking about it."

In this first stage, you are thinking about change and becoming motivated to get started.

You might be in this stage if you

- have been considering change but are not quite ready to start
- believe that your health, energy level, or overall well-being will improve if you develop new habits
- are not sure how you will overcome the roadblocks that may keep you from starting to change

Preparation: "I have made up my mind to take action."

In this next stage, you are making plans and

thinking of specific ideas that will work for you.

You might be in this stage if you

- have decided that you are going to change and are ready to take action
- have set some specific goals that you would like to meet
- are getting ready to put your plan into action

Action: "I have started to make changes."

In this third stage, you are acting on your plan and making the changes you set out to achieve.

You might be in this stage if you

- have been making eating, physical activity, and other behavior changes in the last 6 months or so
- are adjusting to how it feels to eat healthier, be more active, and make other changes such as getting more sleep or reducing screen time
- have been trying to overcome things that sometimes block your success

Maintenance: "I have a new routine."

In this final stage, you have become used to your changes and have kept them up for more than 6 months.

You might be in this stage if

- your changes have become a normal part of your routine
- you have found creative ways to stick with your routine
- you have had slip-ups and setbacks but have been able to get past them and make progress

Did you find your stage of change? Read on for ideas about what you can do next.

Contemplation: Are you thinking of making changes?

Making the leap from thinking about change to taking action can be hard and may take time. Asking yourself about the pros (benefits) and cons (things that get in the way) of changing your habits may be helpful. How would life be better if you made some changes?

Think about how the benefits of healthy eating or regular physical activity might relate to your overall health. For example, suppose your blood glucose, also called blood sugar, is a bit high and you have a parent, brother, or sister who has type 2 diabetes. This means you also may develop type 2 diabetes. You may find that it is easier to be physically active and eat healthy knowing that it may help control blood glucose and protect you from a serious disease.

You may learn more about the benefits of changing your eating and physical activity habits from a health care professional. This knowledge may help you take action.

Look at the lists of pros and cons below. Find the items you believe are true for you. Think about factors that are important to you.

Healthy Eating

Pros

- have more energy
- improve my health
- lower my risk for health problems
- maintain a healthy weight
- feel proud of myself
- set an example for friends and family

Cons

- may spend more money and time on food
- may nccd to cook more often at home
- may need to eat less of foods I love
- may need to buy different foods
- may need to convince my family that we all have to eat healthier foods

Physical Activity

Pros	**Cons**
• improve my health	• takes too much time and energy
• reduce my risk for serious health problems	• it is too hot or cold outside
• feel better about myself	• feel self-conscious
• become stronger	• am nervous about my health
• have fun	• could hurt myself
• take time to care for myself	• am not good at being active
• meet new people and spend time with them	• do not know what to do
• have more energy	• have no one to be active with
• maintain a healthy weight	• am not young or fit enough
• become a role model for others	• keeps me from family and friends

Preparation: Have you made up your mind?

If you are in the preparation stage, you are about to take action. To get started, look at your list of pros and cons. How can you make a plan and act on it?

The chart below lists common roadblocks you may face and possible solutions to overcome roadblocks as you begin to change your habits. Think about these things as you make your plan.

Roadblock: I don't have time.

Solution: Make your new healthy habit a priority. Fit in physical activity whenever and wherever you can. Try taking the stairs or getting off the bus a stop early if it is safe to do so. Set aside one grocery shopping day a week, and make healthy meals that you can freeze and eat later when you don't have time to cook.

Roadblock: Healthy habits cost too much.

Solution: You can walk around the mall, a school track, or a local park for free. Eat healthy on a budget by buying in bulk and when items are on sale, and by choosing frozen or canned fruits and vegetables.

Roadblock: I can't make this change alone.

Solution: Recruit others to be active with you, which will help you stay motivated and safe. Consider signing up for a fun fitness class like salsa dancing. Get your family or coworkers on the healthy eating bandwagon. Plan healthy meals together with your family, or start a healthy potluck once a week at work.

Roadblock: I don't like physical activity.

Solution: Forget the old notion that being physically active means lifting weights in a gym. You can be active in many ways, including dancing, walking, or gardening. Make your own list of options that appeal to you. Explore options you never thought about, and stick with what you enjoy.

Roadblock: I don't like healthy foods.

Solution: Try making your old favorite recipes in healthier new ways. For example, you can trim fat from meats and reduce the amount of butter, sugar, and salt you cook with. Use low-fat cheeses or milk rather than whole-milk foods. Add a cup or two of broccoli, carrots, or spinach to casseroles or pasta.

Once you have made up your mind to change your habits, make a plan and set goals for taking action. Here are some ideas for making your plan:

- learn more about healthy eating (https://www.myplate.gov/)
- learn more about being active (see appendix B)
- make lists of
    - healthy foods that you like or may need to eat more of—or more often
    - foods you love that you may need to eat less often
    - things you could do to be more physically active
    - fun activities you like and could do more often, such as dancing

After making your plan, start setting goals for putting your plan into action. Start with small changes. For example, "I'm going to walk for 10 minutes, three times a week." What is the one step you can take right away?

Action: Have you started to make changes?

You are making real changes to your lifestyle, which is fantastic! To stick with your new habits

- review your plan
- look at the goals you set and how well you are meeting them
- overcome roadblocks by planning ahead for setbacks
- reward yourself for your hard work

Track your progress

- Tracking your progress helps you spot your strengths, find areas where you can improve, and stay on course. Record not only what you did, but how you felt while doing it—your feelings can play a role in making your new habits stick.
- Recording your progress may help you stay focused and catch setbacks in meeting your goals. Remember that a setback does not mean you have failed. All of us experience setbacks. The key is to get back on track as soon as you can.
- You can track your progress with online tools such as the NIH Body Weight Planner (https://www.youtube.com/watch?v=v1gluQwi eog). The NIH Body Weight Planner lets you tailor your calorie and physical activity plans to reach your personal goals within a specific time period.

Overcome roadblocks

- Remind yourself why you want to be healthier. Perhaps you want the energy to play with your nieces and nephews or to be able to carry your own grocery bags. Recall your reasons for making changes when slip-ups occur. Decide to take the first step to get back on track.

- Problem-solve to "outsmart" roadblocks. For example, plan to walk indoors, such as at a mall, on days when bad weather keeps you from walking outside.
- Ask a friend or family member for help when you need it, and always try to plan ahead. For example, if you know that you will not have time to be physically active after work, go walking with a coworker at lunch or start your day with an exercise video.

Reward yourself

- After reaching a goal or milestone, allow for a nonfood reward such as new workout gear or a new workout device. Also consider posting a message on social media to share your success with friends and family.
- Choose rewards carefully. Although you should be proud of your progress, keep in mind that a high-calorie treat or a day off from your activity routine are not the best rewards to keep you healthy.
- Pat yourself on the back. When negative thoughts creep in, remind yourself how much good you are doing for your health by moving more and eating healthier.

Maintenance: Have you created a new routine?

Make your future a healthy one. Remember that eating healthy, getting regular physical activity, and other healthy habits are lifelong behaviors, not one-time events. Always keep an eye on your efforts and seek ways to deal with the planned and unplanned changes in life.

Now that healthy eating and regular physical activity are part of your routine, keep things interesting, avoid slip-ups, and find ways to cope with what life throws at you.

Add variety and stay motivated

Mix up your routine with new physical activities and goals, physical activity buddies, foods, recipes, and rewards.

Deal with unexpected setbacks

Plan ahead to avoid setbacks. For example, find other ways to be active in case of bad weather, injury, or other issues that arise. Think of ways to eat healthy when traveling or dining out, like packing healthy snacks while on the road or sharing an entrée with a friend in a restaurant.

If you do have a setback, don't give up. Setbacks happen to everyone. Regroup and focus on meeting your goals again as soon as you can.

Challenge yourself!

Revisit your goals and think of ways to expand them. For example, if you are comfortable walking 5 days a week, consider adding strength training twice a week. If you have limited your saturated fat intake by eating less fried foods, try cutting back on added sugars, too. Small changes can lead to healthy habits worth keeping.

**When The Going Gets Tough,
Put One Foot in Front of The
Other and Just Keep Going.
Don't Give Up!**

Appendix B: How to Stay Active

Note: Always consult your physician before making any changes to your diet, physical activity or life style.

Physical activity may seem hard if you're overweight. You may get short of breath or tired quickly. Finding or affording the right clothes and equipment may be frustrating. Or, perhaps you may not feel comfortable working out in front of others.

The good news is you can overcome these challenges. Not only can you be active at any size, you can have fun and feel good at the same time.

Can anyone be active?

Research strongly shows that physical activity is safe for almost everyone. The health benefits of physical activity far outweigh the risks.

The activities discussed here are safe for most people. If you have problems moving or staying steady on your feet, or if you get out of breath easily, talk with a health care professional before you start. You also should talk with a health care professional if you are unsure of your health, have any concerns that physical activity may be unsafe for you, or have

- a chronic disease such as diabetes, high blood pressure, or heart disease
- a bone or joint problem—for example, in your back, knee, or hip—that could get worse if you change your physical activity level

Why should I be active?

Being active may help you live longer and protect you from developing serious health problems, such as type 2 diabetes, heart disease, stroke, and certain types of cancer. Regular physical activity is linked to many health benefits, such as

- lower blood pressure and blood glucose, or blood sugar
- healthy bones, muscles, and joints
- a strong heart and lungs
- better sleep at night and improved mood

The Physical Activity Guidelines for Americans define regular physical activity as at least 150 minutes a week of moderate-intensity aerobic activity, such as brisk walking. Brisk walking is a pace of 3 miles per hour or faster. A moderate-intensity activity makes you breathe harder but does not overwork or overheat you. You should also do muscle-strengthening activities at least 2 days a week.

You may reach this goal by starting with 5 minutes

of physical activity several times a day, 5 to 6 days a week. You could then gradually work up to 10 minutes per session, 3 times a day. If you do even more activity, you may gain even more health benefits.

When combined with healthy eating, regular physical activity may also help you control your weight. However, research shows that even if you can't lose weight or maintain your weight loss, you still can enjoy important health benefits from regular physical activity.

Physical activity also can be a lot of fun if you do activities you enjoy and are active with other people. Being active with others may give you a chance to meet new people or spend more time with family and friends. You also may inspire and motivate one another to get and stay active.

What do I need to know about becoming active?

Choosing physical activities that match your fitness level and health goals can help you stay motivated and keep you from getting hurt. You may feel some minor discomfort or muscle soreness when you first become active. These feelings should go away as you get used to your activity. However, if you feel sick to your stomach or have pain, you may have done too much. Go easier and then slowly build up your activity level. Some activities, such as walking or swimming, are less likely to cause injuries.

If you have been inactive, start slowly and see how you feel. Gradually increase how long and how often you are active. If you need guidance, check with a health care or certified fitness professional.

Here are some tips for staying safe during physical activity:

- Wear the proper safety gear, such as a bike helmet if you are bicycling.
- Make sure any sports equipment you use works and fits properly.
- Look for safe places to be active. For instance, walk in well-lit areas where other people are around. Be active with a friend or group.
- Stay hydrated to replace the body fluids you lose through sweating and to prevent you from getting overheated.
- If you are active outdoors, protect yourself from the sun with sunscreen and a hat or protective visor and clothing.
- Wear enough clothing to keep warm in cold or windy weather. Layers are best.

If you don't feel right, stop your activity. If you have any of the following warning signs, stop and seek help right away:

- pain, tightness, or pressure in your chest or neck, shoulder, or arm
- extreme shortness of breath
- dizziness or sickness

Check with a health care professional about what to do if you have any of these warning signs. If your activity is causing pain in your joints, feet, ankles, or legs, you also should consult a health care professional to see if you may need to change the type or amount of activity you are doing.

What kinds of activities can I do?

You don't need to be an athlete or have special skills or equipment to make physical activity part of your life. Many types of activities you do every day, such as walking your dog or going up and down steps at home or at work, may help improve your health.

Try different activities you enjoy. If you like an activity, you're more likely to stick with it. Anything that gets you moving around, even for a few minutes at a time, is a healthy start to getting fit.

Walking

Walking is free and easy to do—and you can do it

almost anywhere. Walking will help you

- burn calories
- improve your fitness
- lift your mood
- strengthen your bones and muscles

If you are concerned about safety, try walking in a shopping mall or park where it is well lit and other people are around. Many malls and parks have benches where you can take a quick break. Walking with a friend or family member is safer than walking alone and may provide the social support you need to meet your activity goals.

If you don't have time for a long walk, take several short walks instead. For example, instead of a 30-minute walk, add three 10-minute walks to your day. Shorter spurts of activity are easier to fit into a busy schedule.

Walking tips

- Wear comfortable, well-fitting walking shoes with a lot of support, and socks that absorb sweat.
- Dress for the weather if you are walking outdoors. In cold weather, wear layers of clothing you can remove if you start getting too warm. In hot weather, protect yourself against the sun and heat.

- Warm up by walking more slowly for the first few minutes. Cool down by slowing your pace.

Dancing

Dancing can be a lot of fun while it tones your muscles, strengthens your heart and lungs, and boosts your mood. You can dance at a health club, dance studio, or even at home. Just turn on some lively music and start moving. You also can dance to a video on your TV or computer.

If you have trouble standing on your feet for a long time, try dancing while sitting down. Chair dancing lets you move your arms and legs to music while taking the weight off your feet.

Bicycling

Riding a bicycle spreads your weight among your arms, back, and hips. For outdoor biking, you may want to try a mountain bike. Mountain bikes have wider tires and are sturdier than bikes with thinner tires. You can buy a larger seat to make biking more comfortable.

For indoor biking, you may want to try a recumbent bike. On this type of bike, you sit lower to the ground with your legs reaching forward to the pedals. Your body is in more of a reclining position, which may feel better than sitting straight up. The seat on a recumbent bike is also wider than the seat on a regular bike.

If you decide to buy a bike, check how much weight it can support to make sure it is safe for you.

Workout clothing tips

- Clothes made of fabrics that absorb sweat are best for working out.
- Comfortable, lightweight clothes allow you to move more easily.
- Tights or spandex shorts are the best bottoms to wear to prevent inner-thigh chafing.
- Women should wear a bra that provides extra support during physical activity.

Water workouts

Swimming and water workouts put less stress on your joints than walking, dancing, or biking. If your feet, back, or joints hurt when you stand, water activities may be best for you. If you feel self-conscious about wearing a bathing suit, you can wear shorts and a T-shirt while you swim.

Exercising in water

- Lets you be more flexible. You can move your body in water in ways you may not be able to on land.

- Reduces your risk of hurting yourself. Water provides a natural cushion, which keeps you from pounding or jarring your joints.
- Helps prevent sore muscles.
- Keeps you cool, even when you are working hard.

You don't need to know how to swim to work out in water. You can do shallow- or deep-water exercises at either end of the pool without swimming. For instance, you can do laps while holding onto a kickboard and kicking your feet. You also can walk or jog across the width of the pool while moving your arms.

For shallow-water workouts, the water level should be between your waist and chest. During deep-water workouts, most of your body is underwater. For safety and comfort, wear a foam belt or life jacket.

Tips for protecting your hair

If you're worried that pool water will damage or mess up your hair, try these tips:

- Use a swim cap to help protect your hair from pool chemicals and getting wet.
- Wear a natural hairstyle, short braids, locs, or twists, which may be easier to style after a water workout.

- Buy a shampoo to remove chlorine buildup, available at most drug stores, if your hair feels dry or damaged after a pool workout.

Strength training

Strength training involves using free weights, weightlifting machines, resistance bands, or your own body weight to make your muscles stronger. Lower-body strength training will improve your balance and prevent falls.

Strength training may help you

- build and maintain strong muscles as you get older
- continue to perform activities of daily living, such as carrying groccrics or moving furniture
- keep your bones strong, which may help prevent osteoporosis and fractures

If you are just starting out, using a weightlifting machine may be safer than dumbbells. As you get fit, you may want to add free-weight exercises with dumbbells.

You do not need a weight bench or large dumbbells to do strength training at home. You can use a pair of hand weights to do bicep curls. You can also use your own body weight: for example, get up and down from a chair.

Proper form is very important when lifting weights. You may hurt yourself if you don't lift weights properly. You may want to schedule a session with a certified fitness professional to learn which exercises to do and how to do them safely. Check with your health insurer about whether your health plan covers these services.

If you decide to buy a home gym, check how much weight it can support to make sure it is safe for you.

Strength-training tips

- Aim for at least 2 days per week of strengthen-training activities.
- Try to perform each exercise 8 to 12 times. If that's too hard, the weight you are lifting is too heavy. If it's too easy, your weight is too light.
- Try to exercise all the major muscle groups. These groups include the muscles of the legs, hips, chest, back, abdomen, shoulders, and arms.
- Don't work the same muscles 2 days in a row. Your muscles need time to recover.

Mind and body exercise

Your local hospital or fitness, recreation, or community center may offer classes such as yoga, tai chi, or Pilates. You also may find some of these workouts online and can download them to a computer, smart phone, or other device. These types of activities may help you

- become stronger and more flexible
- feel more relaxed
- improve balance and posture

Your local hospital or fitness, recreation, or community center may offer classes such as yoga, tai chi, or Pilates.

These classes also can be a lot of fun and add variety to your workout routine. If some movements are hard to do or you have injuries you are concerned about, talk with the instructor about how to adapt the exercises and poses to meet your needs—or start with a beginner's class.

Daily life activities

Daily life activities, such as cleaning out the attic or washing the car, are great ways to get moving. Small changes can add more physical activity to your day and improve your health. Try these:

- Take 2- to 3-minute walking breaks at work several times a day, if possible.
- Stand, walk, or stretch in place during TV commercials.
- Take the stairs instead of the elevator or escalator whenever you can.

- Park farther from where you are going and walk the rest of the way.

Even a shopping trip can be exercise because it provides a chance to walk and carry your bags. Chores such as mowing the lawn, raking leaves, and gardening also count.

Where can I be active?

You can find many fun places to be active. Having more than one place may keep you from getting bored. Here are some options:

- Join or take a class at a local fitness, recreation, or community center.
- Enjoy the outdoors by taking a hike or going for a walk in a safe local park, neighborhood, or mall.
- Work out in the comfort of your own home with a workout video or by finding a fitness channel on your TV, tablet, or other mobile device.

Tips for choosing a fitness center

- Make sure the center has exercise equipment for people who weigh more and staff to show you how to use it.
- Ask if the center has any special classes for people just starting out, older adults, or people with mobility or health issues.

- See if you can try out the center or take a class before you join.
- Try to find a center close to work or home. The quicker and easier the center is to get to, the better your chances of using it often.
- Make sure you understand the rules for joining and ending your membership, what your membership fee covers, any related costs, and the days and hours of operation.

How can I get past my roadblocks?

You most likely will face roadblocks that keep you from meeting your physical activity goals. Think about what keeps you from being active, then try to come up with creative ways to address those roadblocks. Here are a few examples to help you get started:

Barrier: I don't have enough time.

Solution: Instead of doing one long workout session, build in three 10-minute bursts of activity during your day, such as a brisk walk. Even standing up instead of sitting at your desk has benefits.

Barrier: I just don't like exercise.

Solution: Good news! You don't have to run a marathon or go to the gym all the time to benefit from being active. To make physical activity more fun, try something you enjoy doing, such as dancing to the radio or taking a yoga class with friends. Many people find they start to like exercise better the more they do it.

Barrier: I'm worried about my health or getting hurt.

Solution: If you have a hard time being active because of your health, talk with a health care professional first. A certified fitness professional can also guide you on how to be active safely.

Barrier: I feel self-conscious working out in front of others.

Solution: Start being active at home until you feel more confident. Be active with friends who will support and encourage you.

How can I stick with my physical activity plan?

Sticking with a plan to be physically active can be a challenge. Online tools such as the NIH Body Weight Planner (https://www.youtube.com/watch?v=v1gluQwieog) can help. The NIH Body Weight Planner lets you tailor your calorie and physical activity plans to reach your personal goals within a specific time period.

You also can download fitness apps that let you enter information to track your progress using a computer or smart phone or other mobile device.

Devices you can wear, such as pedometers and fitness trackers, may help you count steps, calories, and minutes of physical activity. Trackers can help you set goals and monitor progress. You wear most of these devices on your wrist like a watch, or clipped to your clothing.

Keeping an activity journal is another good way to help you stay motivated and on track to reach your fitness goals.

Set goals. As you track your activity, try to set specific short- and long-term goals. For example, instead of "I will be more active," set a goal such as "I will take a walk after lunch at least 2 days a week." Getting started with a doable goal is a good way to form a new habit. A short-term goal may be to walk 5 to 10 minutes, 5 days a week. A long-term goal may be to do at least 150 minutes of moderate-intensity physical activity a week.

Get support. Ask a family member or friend to be active with you. Your workout buddy can help make your activities more fun and can cheer you on and help you meet your goals.

Track progress. You may not feel as though you

are making progress, but when you look back at where you started, you may be pleasantly surprised. Making regular activity part of your life is a big step. Start slowly and praise yourself for every goal you set and achieve.

Review your goals. Did you meet your goals? If not, why? Are they doable? Did you hit a roadblock trying to meet your goal? What will you do differently next week? Brainstorm some options to overcome future roadblocks. Ask a friend or family member to help support your goals.

Pick nonfood rewards. Whether your goal is to be active 15 minutes a day, to walk farther than you did last week, or simply to stay positive, recognizing your efforts is an important part of staying on track. Decide how you will reward yourself. Some ideas for rewards include getting new music to charge you up or buying new workout gear.

Be patient with yourself. Don't get discouraged if you have setbacks from time to time. If you can't achieve your goal the first time or can only stick to your goals for part of the week, remind yourself that this is all part of establishing new habits.

Look ahead. Try to focus on what you will do differently moving forward, rather than on what went wrong. Pat yourself on the back for trying.

Most importantly, don't give up. Any movement, even for a short time, is a good thing. Each activity you add to your life is another step toward a healthier you.